Contents

An Epidemiological Alert was issued by the WHO and the Pan American Health Organization in May 2015 when the Zika virus was reported in Brazil. Prior to 2015, Zika virus caused outbreaks in areas of Africa and Southeast Asia. Since May 2015, more than a million people have been infected in Brazil, and the Brazilian government has announced that there has been a 20% rise in cases of microcephaly in new-born babies.

Between May 2015 and January 2016, Zika virus has spread to much of South America; the Caribbean; Samoa in the Pacific Islands, and Cape Verde in Africa.

Why should pregnant women, or those thinking about having a baby, be especially vigilant? What can people do to keep the mosquitoes that carry the virus away from themselves and their children? This book will explain what the Zika virus is; where it came from; and, most importantly, what steps people can take to avoid catching the virus.

Chapter 1:   What is Zika virus?

Prior to its first major outbreak in 2007, few people had heard of the Zika virus. Scientists knew of its existence as it had appeared in 1947 in Uganda, Africa. In April 1947, six platforms were placed in the forest canopy in the Zika Forest near Entebbe. On each platform was placed a cage containing a Rhesus monkey, and scientists from the East African Virus Research Institute in Entebbe were hoping to discover more about Yellow fever in the hope that the monkeys would be bitten by mosquitoes.

The first monkey developed a fever that lasted for a month. A sample of the monkey's blood was injected into mice who did not develop any illness. The second monkey did not have a fever, but an unknown virus was grown in the laboratory from its blood. Mice were injected with the virus, and some became paralysed, and one mouse died. One of the other monkey cages caused great alarm when it was taken down from the platform: a large python had entered the cage when the snake was slim, and having eaten the poor monkey, became so fat that it could not get out again.

The unknown virus was named Zika after the forest in which it was first discovered. Zika is an arbovirus (a flavivirus from the family Flaviviridae) that is related to other viruses such as Dengue fever, Yellow fever, Japanese Encephalitis and West Nile Virus. The diseases are transmitted to humans by mosquitoes and ticks: arbovirus means 'borne by arthropods'. Zika virus (ZIKV) was first isolated in a human in Nigeria in 1954. It surfaced a number of times in Africa and and then Southeast Asia, and was known to cause a flu-like illness that was generally not fatal. The mosquito *Aedes aegypti* is known to be the carrier of the virus.

In April 2007, there was a major outbreak of Zika virus on the Pacific island of Yap, where three-quarters of the population (out of 10,000) became ill, although it only seemed to occur in people over the age of three. The illness caused a rash, conjunctivitis, arthralgia (aching joints), headache, and sometimes severe pain behind the eyes, and an upset stomach. However, a lot of people who are infected with ZIKV do not have any symptoms at all, and it only shows up when a blood test is done.

By 2013, ZIKV had reached Tahiti. A man developed flu-like symptoms of a raised temperature and joint pains: he did not seek medical attention as he thought that the fever would soon abate. Two weeks later he felt ill again, and thought that the flu had returned. Again, he did not seek medical assistance, but a further two weeks later he finally went to see his doctor as he had blood in his semen, and he then tested positive for ZIKV. This case raised the possibility that ZIKV could be sexually transmitted. A second case involved a man who had been infected in Senegal in Africa. He returned home to the United States where he too discovered blood in his semen, and his wife went on to develop ZIKV. It is suspected that the virus could also be in other bodily fluids.

Other parts of French Polynesia were also affected in 2013, with around 28,000 people infected. By 2014, the virus had reached New Caledonia and the Cook Islands. In 2015 the virus reached Easter Island, and then mainland South America where it appeared in Brazil.

Zika virus affected northeast Brazil in May 2015, and since then it has spread to most states of the country. Brazil has been badly affected by the virus, with an estimated one million and a half people infected. Those worst affected are pregnant women, as a much higher than average number of babies have been born with microcephaly: this is a condition where the head of a baby is abnormally small because the brain has not developed properly. The children are left with developmental delays, learning difficulties, and a shortened life-span. Microcephaly is diagnosed when the head is below average size, with the head circumference measuring less than 31.5 - 32 cm at birth. There were fewer than 150 cases in Brazil during the whole of 2014, but there have been more than 4,000 reported cases since May 2014 to January 2016.

Zika virus has also caused other neurological conditions in adults.

Chapter 2: How is Zika virus caught?

Zika virus is caught when a person is bitten by an infected *Aedes aegypti* mosquito: it is thought that other species of *Aedes* mosquito may also transmit ZIKV, but it has not yet been proved. If an uninfected mosquito bites a person already infected with ZIKV, the virus enters the mosquito and multiplies. Within two weeks the mosquito can then transmit the virus by biting more people.

ZIKV cannot be caught unless a person is bitten by an *Aedes aegypti* mosquito that is already infected. It may also be possible to acquire ZIKV through having sex with an infected person: the virus has been identified in the semen and urine of two infected men, but it is not known whether it can be transmitted to another person in bodily fluids, like the Ebola virus. It is believed that a small number of people may have been infected via sexual transmission.

Pregnant mothers can be infected at any time during the pregnancy, and it appears that the mother may be able to transmit the virus to their unborn babies. The virus may cause still birth or birth defects. There has been a marked increase in the number of babies born with microcephaly in Brazil. There has also been a marked rise in the number of people with neurological conditions like Guillain-Barre Syndrome.

Guillain-Barre Syndrome, or GBS, can result from a number of viral and bacteriological infections. GBS causes weakness, tingling sensations, and sometimes paralysis in the arms, legs or upper body. In severe cases, paralysis of the chest muscles can result in the sufferer having to breathe via a ventilator. Most people eventually recover from GBS.

The symptoms of Zika virus are a rash; a fever; headache; sometimes mild swelling of the hands or feet; muscle pain; joint pain; conjunctivitis and pain behind the eyes. Many people do not have any symptoms at all, and the virus only shows up in a blood test investigating another disease. There have been no deaths reported that have been due to Zika virus infection.

There is no antiviral treatment for the Zika virus. Rest and painkillers are recommended by clinicians, with antihistamines if the rash causes pruritus. People with confirmed ZIKV should drink lots of fluids to replace that lost by sweating, and possibly vomiting.

Chapter 3: Which countries are affected by Zika virus?

The Centers for Disease Control and the World Health Organization are monitoring the developing situation closely as cases are reported around the world. At the time of writing, cases are being reported outside of South America, usually the result of travelers returning home from infected areas.

Zika has been confirmed by the CDC in the following countries:

Americas

Barbados
Bolivia
Brazil
Colombia
Dominican Republic
Ecuador
El Salvador
French Guiana
Guadeloupe
Guatemala
Guyana
Haiti

Honduras
Martinique
Mexico
Panama
Paraguay
Puerto Rico
Saint Martin
Suriname
US Virgin Islands
Venezuela

Oceania/ Pacific Islands

Samoa

Africa

Cape Verde

Countries with reported cases of Zika in returning travelers:

Australia
Denmark
Germany
Sweden
Thailand
United Kingdom

United States: Arkansas, California, Florida, Hawaii, Illinois, Massachusetts, Minnesota, New Jersey, New York, Oregon, Texas, Virginia and the District of Columbia

More countries are expected to report the infection in more returning travelers. The WHO predicts that ZIKV "will eventually end up in virtually every Western Hemisphere country". It was reported on 28 January 2016 that *Aedes aegypti* mosquitoes have been seen on the Kent coast and around Chichester in Sussex, in southern England.

It is predicted that climate change could worsen the spread of Zika virus and other infectious diseases as mosquitoes and other insects prefer warmer climates. Heat makes mosquitoes breed faster, and they will intrude further and further into northern and southern temperate zones. The mosquitoes will live longer and bite people more frequently.

Dr. Margaret Chan, director-general of the WHO, has warned that El Nino's weather patterns in 2016 are expected to greatly increase mosquito populations in many areas.

The mosquito *Aedes aegypti* that is causing Zita virus prefers to feed on human blood, and it breeds close to human populations in small pools of water like ditches, water butts, garden ponds, and empty cans and bottles. Construction sites are a magnet for mosquitoes as there are often holes full of rainwater that are prime breeding grounds for them. *Aedes aegypti* live for one to two months, and can have many offspring in that time. The female lays around 300 eggs.

And 390 million people are infected with the Dengue virus each year, largely as a result of bites from *Aedes aegypti.*

Chapter 4: How are countries preparing to tackle Zika virus?

Pregnant women are being advised not to travel to regions affected by the Zika virus. Airlines are beginning to offer refunds to passengers who have booked flights to countries affected by the virus. Thus far, British Airways have stated that pregnant customers with flights booked to Sao Paulo and Rio de Janeiro in Brazil, and Mexico City and Cancun in Mexico can change their bookings without charge, or delay their journey or choose an alternative destination. This applies until the end of February 2016. American Airlines will provide pregnant passengers with a full refund if they have documentation from their healthcare provider, and if they were to travel to San Salvador in El Salvador; San Pedro Sula and Tegucigalpa in Honduras; Panama City or Guatemala City. United Airlines has said that it will allow customers worried about the Zika virus to cancel or postpone their flights if they were to travel to affected areas.

People who have returned from visits to areas affected by ZIKV should see their healthcare providers, especially if they have developed flu-like symptoms since their return. Pregnant women with diagnoses of Zika virus are advised to have ultrasounds every 3 - 4 weeks to monitor the baby's growth.

US health officials have issued guidelines for the care of babies born to mothers who traveled or lived in areas affected by Zika during their pregnancies. For infants without microcephaly but whose mothers received a positive or inconclusive test for ZIKV, should be tested for the virus.

With the summer months to come in the northern hemisphere, scientists are concerned about the possible spread of the Zika virus. President Obama has called for urgent action against the virus, with the rapid development of a new testing kit to quickly identify Zika infection.

Brazil's government is deploying 220,000 soldiers to go from house to house handing out leaflets advising people on how to eradicate the mosquitoes causing the virus, and how to avoid being bitten by a mosquito. *Aedes aegypti* mosquitoes typically bite people during the day, and also around dawn and dusk. People should use mosquito repellent containing DEET on areas not covered by clothing, and not leave anything outside their homes that could collect standing water, like old tyres.

The Pan American Health Organization (part of the WHO) issued an Epidemiological Alert in May 2015, and it advised prevention and control measures like eliminating mosquito breeding sites by houses, schools, parks, and anywhere accessed by the public. Families should spray their homes with insecticide to deter mosquitoes.

The UK and other European countries already have surveillance techniques in place at seaports, airports, the premises of used tyre importers, and motorway service stations. There have been ongoing outbreaks of West Nile Virus in southern and eastern Europe; Chikungunya fever in France and Italy; Dengue fever in Madeira, Croatia and France, and Vivax malaria in Greece, which has resulted in strategies being in place to hopefully deal with any incursions of the mosquito *Aedes aegypti*.

Public Health England have urged men in the UK to wear condoms for a month when having sex after returning from any of the 23 countries affected by the Zika virus.

Campaigners are calling on Latin American governments to rethink their policies on contraception and abortion because of the spread of Zika virus, which they fear will lead to a rise in women's deaths from unsafe abortions as well as the predicted surge in babies with microcephaly.

The governments of Colombia, El Salvador and Ecuador have advised women to postpone getting pregnant for up to two years, which reproductive health groups say is impossible in countries where birth control is not easily available and many women fall pregnant through sexual violence.

The burden of Ebola virus fell mainly on women in Africa as mothers and as care-givers, and the same situation will possibly happen to the women of South America.

Chapter 5: How to control the *Aedes aegypti* mosquito

The search for a safe vaccine is under way, but it could take anything from three to ten years before one would be ready to be used. Scientists are already warning that the virus has mutated and become more virulent. In the meantime, what is to be done? Controlling the mosquitoes, with the target of eradicating them would be the ultimate goal, ending the scourge of mosquito-spread diseases.

One method that had proved to be successful is the Sterile Insect Technique, or SIT. This method was used in the 1950s, and worked by dosing male mosquitoes with radiation. The process leaves the irradiated males feeling and looking very sickly, and the females do not want to mate with them, leading to a massive fall in mosquito numbers. The SIT was used to successfully eradicate screw-worm in North America, and the Tsetse Fly in Zanzibar.

Another extremely successful method is to use genetically modified mosquitoes to dramatically reduce their population. *Aedes aegypti* has spread around the world by hitching rides in shipping containers, used tyres, and anything that provides a suitable nesting site for the mosquito's eggs. Biotechnology company Oxitec has created genetically modified male mosquitoes that mate with wild females, who then produce sterile offspring. A pilot programme in Brazil used genetically modified male *Aedes aegypti* mosquitoes and successfully reduced the local population by 80%. Oxitec are already releasing self-limiting male mosquitoes in a suburb of Sao Paulo.

This method of controlling the *Aedes aegypti* mosquito seems far more sensible than telling women to put off becoming pregnant until 2018, as suggested by public health officials in El Salvador. Why 2018? Does the date have some significance?

Chapter 6: How to avoid being bitten by the *Aedes aegypti* mosquito

The CDC has advised that insect repellents, when used as directed by the manufacturer, are safe and effective for everyone, including pregnant and nursing women. Most insect repellents can be safely used on children, but do not used products containing oil of lemon eucalyptus on children under 3 years of age, and be careful that older children do not get the oil on their hands as they might rub it on their eyes and cause irritation. Repellents containing DEET, picaridin, IR3535, and some para-menthane-diol products provide long-lasting protection against mosquitoes. Do not use insect repellent under clothing as it will not work efficiently. Apply sunscreen before insect repellent. Treat clothing with permethrin, or purchase permethrin-treated clothing.

The CDC advises that long-sleeved shirts, and trousers rather than shorts should be worn whenever the weather permits. Air conditioning and window and door screens keep mosquitoes out of the house. In hotels always empty standing water out of buckets and flower pots.

The Millennium Summit Meeting of the United Nations in 2000 resulted in the UN Millennium Declaration. Target 6C of the Millennium Development Goals aimed to have halted by 2015, and begun to reverse the incidence of malaria and other major diseases by providing insecticide-treated mosquito nets to all children under the age of 5, with the aim of eradicating mosquito-borne diseases. The Millennium Development Goals Report 2015 stated that more than 900 million insecticide-treated mosquito nets were delivered to malaria-endemic countries in sub-Saharan Africa between 2004 and 2014. That so much has been done is admirable, and now ALL children under the age of 5, living with the threat of diseases such as Zika virus should be given a mosquito net by the United Nations, or by their country's governments. Prevention using a cheap bed-net is much less costly than having to treat sick children and their families.

The great researcher of infectious diseases, Robert S. Desowitz, advised that in his opinion, one of the cheapest and most effective deterrents against mosquito bites was the humble mosquito net. Used properly so that the net covers the whole of the bed down to the floor, and fine enough to keep out mosquitoes, flies and other biting insects, and not against the skin so that a mosquito can bite through it, is the best deterrent.

The 2016 Summer Olympic Games are to be held in Rio de Janeiro, Brazil in August. The organisers of the Games are committed to daily inspections, before and during the Games, of the Olympic venues to remove stagnant water where mosquitoes could breed. The Games will be during Brazil's dry season, when hopefully there will be a smaller population of mosquitoes.

Dr Margaret Chan, director-general of the World Health Organization, has stated that Zika has gone "from a mild threat to one of alarming proportions". Up to four million cases are predicted in the Americas in 2016.

At the moment, all that governments seem able to do is to advise women not to get pregnant during the Zika outbreak. American scientists searching for a vaccine have warned that it will be at least ten years before one is safe to use. With no vaccine yet in sight, controlling mosquitoes is vital, and pressure must be kept on all authorities, whether at the local or international level, to fund mosquito-elimination programmes.

In 1992, the English writer PD James wrote a book called 'The Children of Men' about a growing infertility problem of humankind that leads to just one child about to be born in the whole world. At the time it seemed simply a work of fiction, but the Zika virus could perhaps make that an all too terrifying reality if it continues to spread around the world.

Select bibliography

CDC   Zika virus   23 January 2016

Brazil's president declares war on mosquitoes to slow spread of Zika virus. *Reuters*. 27 January 2016

Butler, Anne. Zika virus found in Australian travelers returning from South America. *ABC Australia*. 26 January 2016

Harvey, Chelsea. How climate change could worsen the spread of Zika virus and other infectious diseases. *The Washington Post*. 26 January 2016

Desowitz, Robert S. 1991. *The malaria papers: more tales of parasites and people, research and reality.* WW Norton, New York

Millennium Summit of the United Nations. New York. 2000 *UN Millennium Declaration*. Target 6C: Have halved by 2015 and begun to reverse the incidence of malaria and other major diseases: Proportion of children under 5 sleeping under insecticide-treated bed nets

Desowitz, Robert S. 1997. *Tropical diseases from 50,000 BC to 2500 AD.* HarperCollins, London

CDC   Health advisory.   Recognising, managing, and reporting Zika virus infections in travelers returning from Central America, South America, the Caribbean, and Mexico. 15 January 2016

How to control Zika. *Oxitec.com/oxitec-video,* 2016

Schaffner, Francis...[et al] 2013. Development of guidelines for the surveillance of invasive mosquitoes in Europe. *Parasites & Vectors.* Vol.6:209

Pan   American   Health   Organization Epidemiological Alert: Zika virus infection. 7 May 2015

Vaux, Alexander GC and Medlock, Jolyon M. 2015. Current status of invasive mosquito surveillance in the UK.   *Parasites & Vectors.* Vol.8:351

Zika virus. *Public Health England.*   11 December 2015

Chatterjee, Pritha. Microcephaly in Brazil showed a 20% jump in cases. *The Indian Express*. 26 January 2016

Gallagher, James. Zika virus: up to four million Zika cases predicted. *BBC News*. 28 January 2016

Fernandez, Colin. Mosquitoes linked to baby defect are in UK. *Daily Mail* 29 January 2016

Public Health England. Men in the UK are being urged to wear condoms for a month after returning from any of the 23 countries affected by the Zika virus. *Sky News*. 29 January 2016

Boseley, Sarah and Douglas, Bruce. Zika outbreak raises fears of rise in deaths from unsafe abortions. *The Guardian*. 29 January 2016